CONTENTS

ACHIEVE THE HAPPINESS
AND FREEDOM YOU DESERVE IN 1 YEAR

OCD

FREEDOM

FORMULA

A workbook that contains an
unmatched *2-STEP* healing system that
will finally make you breakfree from
your mental prison

STEVEN PAUL

CHAPTER 1

INTRODUCTION

Listen, whoever decided to get access to this book, I congratulate you, and I assure you that you will see a massive difference in you and your life.

This book is specially designed for people with severe OCD.

I laid out the core principle of almost everything related to OCD.

In addition, I have not included any rubbish talks in this book, I know in many books most of the content is filled with stuff that's unnecessary just to make the book big in size.

This won't be the case here. All the lines and all the content are pure gold. You won't even need a highlighter.

I focused this book on quality, not on unnecessary quantity.

To get the best out of this book 'Follow my advice blindly'- at the beginning, it won't or might not make sense but in the end, you'll see the whole picture.

Entrust yourself to me.

Give this book a year.

And you my friend will see a huge difference and real happiness in your life.

This book is like an optimized workout plan for you.

I personally had to go through 80% crap research. Making myself go through all kinds of medications and therapies like ERP, CBT, Hypnotherapy you name it and all sorts of trial and error and experiments with me, to get the remaining 10-20% gold strategies that worked.

You, my friend, saved lots of time, energy, and frustration by giving yourself chance to get access to this book.

Congratulations.

You have no idea what's waiting for you.

Get ready to change your reality.

And I say this again *"Follow this book like a holy grail and change your reality forever"*.

CHAPTER 2

MY STORY

I will keep the story short and precise.

I always had OCD from childhood, but it was not that severe, but I realised I use to become upset or sad at small stuff pretty quickly. Go deep with small, small stuff or something that happened with me during a particular day.

But still it was okay, but as I reached my adolescent age and my studies became higher especially from 9th standard as per as I remember, I use to get innate stress while studying, fuck it was so pathetic, hundreds of thoughts running in my mind that started from a single thought I was over-thinking on and on, but still it was not that severe, it gave me depression definitely but still nothing compared to peak point of OCD, I had during my 11th and 12th standards later.

It affected my social life a lot.

My classmates thought I was weird, dumb... some of them use to call me invisible cause it didn't matter I existed or not. I had no influence.

During my 11th standard my depression became more severe, like really severe, at this point I couldn't stand social circle, just wanted to lock myself in a room alone, even though I was alive felt like dying, pressure from society to perform well in studies increased it to another level, and I was not able to perform well at all in studies even though I gave all my will, couldn't concentrate in class nor in practical session, teachers complaining in parent-teacher meet, I felt like I am a disappointment, dumb-ass fuck, felt like hopeless creature on earth.

When I went to doctor for my depression (which I thought was the cause that time), that was when my doctor stated that I had OCD (didn't know what it was back then), they gave me pills which had no effect, only made me feel sleepy.

I only use to sleep in my hostel, basically, all I did was sleep, go to school, come back eat, sleep, repeat, and also it was hard for me to mix with the hostellers.

My life was literally fucked.

So, I went deep on OCD, found all the therapies that were available on the Internet, it came out to be ERP, CBT, and hypnotherapy. I kept these therapies in my mind. And decided to experiment with all of them after my 12th standard.

I was superstitious during that time and too much entrusting myself on God which definitely contributed on my OCD (you will know why in the latter part of the chapter, keynote - I am not putting God in a negative light here, I am just saying believe in yourself more than anyone else). I use to ask God for happiness and curing me of my OCD. But nothing really happened.

The concept of God only gives you temporary relief, but ultimately you have to take action. I find it funny thinking about it now, and I will tell you one thing, more than anyone else trust yourself, believe in yourself, only you can save yourself and make yourself grow and nobody can. Taking the steps to heal yourself, having a belief you will do it, the belief which is coming from yourself and not from an external source that's what makes you stronger.

TAKING THE CORRECT STEPS WITH NO PRAYING IS MUCH BETTER THAN PRAYING AND CRYING WITH NO STEPS.

Now you must be thinking what steps...

Don't worry about the steps. The steps and the process are laid out in the book. The only thing you have to do is to follow it dedicatedly. Just promise - stop asking help from GOD, even God helps those who help themselves. And start believing in yourself which will, in turn, help to strengthen your belief system.

Anyways back to my class 12, in that time I was also superstitious, I tried gemstones, I searched on the internet which gemstones are good for my zodiac sign, gives more positive energy with the concept of stars alignment and constellations and shit. Guess what just a waste of my money and time.

And finally during my 12th final exams, shit hit the fan, I entered the severe OCD mode, couldn't concentrate on my studies, thousands of thoughts running in my mind, at times it felt like million, felt like my head will burst, felt like suicide is the only way to relief.

I was walking to the door and coming back to my study table compulsively, drowning through my thoughts to only realise later that I have been doing this compulsive movement (from door to my table and repeat) almost an hour.

My thoughts jumped from blinking of an eye to the saliva in my mouth, to the walking of my feet, and million other thought-jumps. I covered myself in a blanket, drowned my head inside a pillow. Couldn't eat or sleep (even the pills were not working this time), I reached a point where I couldn't sleep for days and my consciousness became so numb due to lack of sleep that I couldn't understand whether I was living in a dream or reality.

After this horrific experience, I went to another doctor who also gave me pills, but this time the doctor was comparatively understanding, pills that he gave didn't heal me but suppressed it which I needed that time and also made me feel extra hard sleepy. Which I was not complaining, as being awake was more horrific for me.

I knew deep inside pills were not the ultimate solution, so I went for other solutions, the therapies that were on my mind, those were costly but I had no other way, I literally wasted 1000s of bucks, but still unsuccessful except for ERP which was also unsuccessful when it comes to healing but a little helpful, when I say little, I really mean little but still it was a lot for me at that time, like a drop of water for a thirsty guy on a hot desert, like a piece of bread for a poor person who has been hungry for days. The problem with ERP is that there are some tricks and illusion the brain tries to pull at you, that makes you continue the same mental loop, no solution for this in ERP and for multiple mixed OCD as I found for myself to be quite ineffective.

Even after the therapies, didn't heal at all, so I decided to give a gap of a year, cause I knew, I couldn't just do my further studies like the situation I was in.

It got worse and worse, with multiple suicidal thoughts till I reached a point where I gave up and accepted OCD to be a part of my life and let it do whatever it wants to do. Then, something interesting happened; ironically severity of my OCD decreased a little. Not healed though but at least something better than nothing. This epiphany gave me a hope. I slowly but surely started to get the pattern of OCD.

On top of that, I experimented with different mindsets and researched a lot especially on neuroplasticity, putting all the pieces together even from the unsuccessful sessions, with numerous trial and error I got the foolproof system to get healed, when I was on the healing process often times I noticed I use to forget to take the pills, cause I was in a normal mental position and could sleep and perform other activities easily and eventually left my pills cause I was finally happy and was finally free of medication.

Within about a year I was healed to the level I could enjoy my life, control my thoughts, no mental irritation, be social, have cool friends, be in relationship, and most important of all - be happy and free.

CHAPTER 3

HOW TO USE THIS BOOK

So, I welcome you to this chapter...

This chapter is to give you a clear path, on how to use this book.

There are basically two sections:
1. Understanding of Mechanism
2. Application of Mechanism

Understanding of Mechanism includes:

Unit 1: Mechanism of OCD: This unit basically deals with how OCD works, what is it, under which high probability circumstances and behaviour and thinking, it occurred initially.

Unit 2: Mechanism Of Healing: This unit shows the process you have to go through to undergo healing, how to control your mind, exercise and train your unstable mind, strengthening your belief system and key nuances in healing which is slight critical.

Unit 3: Mechanism Of Self-sabotaging: This unit shows certain unconscious, sub-conscious or conscious behaviours that you do that deplete your healing process and how to take care of them and also mention solutions to some key issues.

Application of Mechanism includes:

Unit 4: Summarization of the process: After completing 'Understanding of Mechanism' section, you need to have clear step by step blueprint, so that you don't get overwhelmed, and have a clear direction to achieve your desired freedom and happiness. Also, there are some extra bonus stuff in this unit that will help you in your healing journey.

*note: Don't directly jump to Unit-4, every chapter is related. Start from the beginning and progress sequentially. Otherwise, you would be hurting your own healing process.

Now, let me give you two scenarios:

Scenario 1: I tell you to do a certain workout, say "Bench Press" and you kind of know how to do it, but I am not telling you the proper forms and techniques, and the other key things like grip, variations, range of motion, positioning, mind-muscle connection etc. I am not making you understand the mechanism of the Bench Press exercise.

Scenario 2: A similar scenario where I tell you to do bench press workout but this time, I explain you the forms and techniques, the range of motion, grip and other key stuffs really thoroughly. You get to understand the mechanism of bench press exercise and thus you know how it works and know the dos and the don'ts.

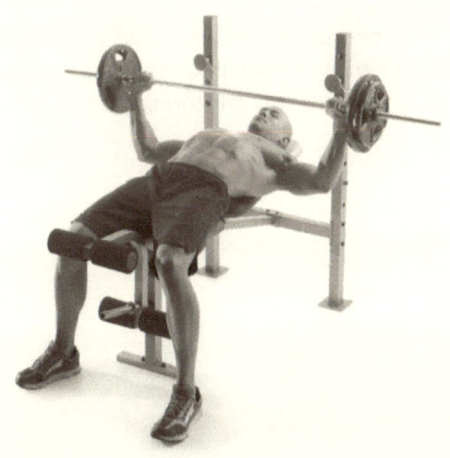

Bench Press Workout

Tell me in which scenario you would do the workout better, obviously in scenario 2. Understanding of mechanism gives you motivation and helps you to understand whether you are on the right track or wrong. Thus, you don't distract yourself or be in confusion what to do and what not to do and as a result of being in the right direction, you achieve your goal.

Therefore, it's my ardent advice that you finish Section-1 first i.e.: Understanding of Mechanism, then proceed to Section- 2 i.e.: Application of Mechanism. *This advice is Mandatory.

Follow the sequence of how I advised you to use this book and you my friend will be healed from OCD and achieve true happiness.

Key-Thing to note:

- If you are under medication, no need to discontinue it, just follow the process laid out in this book along with the medication. Eventually, when you will achieve normal zone quite consistently, you will automatically leave it. Because when the problem exists you remember to take the pill but when the issue disappears it won't even occur in your mind.
- Some lines or words I repeat, because I want to hammer those points into your head because I can't take the chance of you ignoring them.

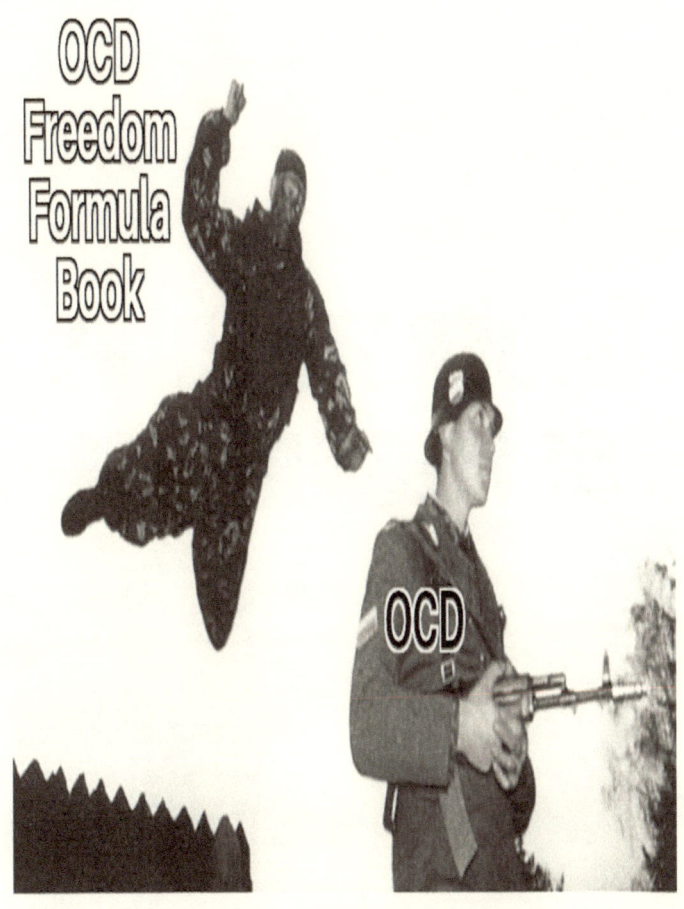

UNDERSTANDING
OF MECHANISM

UNIT 1

MECHANISM
OF OCD

CHAPTER 4

HABIT AND NEUROPLASTICITY

Habit and Neuroplasticity go hand in hand.

Habit is a forming of certain behaviour or skill through repetition subconsciously or consciously.

Neuroplasticity happens when you behave or think in a certain way, or give new information to the brain, new neurons are in formation, with time the wiring of your brain changes from the initial stage and thus you generate certain new behaviour or thinking pattern which becomes subconscious and eventually becomes a habit.

For example: when learning a bicycle, at beginning you were scared, you needed to concentrate on balancing, consistent paddling, looking front etc...., but after a bit of practice it becomes subconscious and effortless.

So, how does it relate to your OCD?

Many people think the change in behaviour or wiring is on the physical level only, but it also happens in the emotional and on the thinking and overall mental level as well.

When you are having certain thinking for a longer period of time, it becomes a habit. An unconscious habit that you lose control over, and the more you try to control it, the more it creates problem.

And thus your thinking affects your behaviour and your behaviour affects your personality.

Let me tell you the general blueprint how in majority people OCD began.

At some point of your life usually in childhood, since the maturity of your mind is like a soft clay, for some reason you start to go deep on certain thought or behaviour consciously or subconsciously, you might or might not be aware of it, and at beginning it didn't cause us any harm, and even it did it was really mild, but again at that moment you were giving new information to your brain, forming new pattern to your thinking, now you slowly started to develop habit of going deep on particular thoughts (you probably wouldn't have, if you knew what consequences it would bring to you), which slowly started to set as permanent – a subconscious habit, habit that is out of your control.

Also, the thing is you are giving unpleasant information to your brain, that's why it's said that small children should always be given freedom, shown love to them, let them play, cause the first 5-7 years of a person is really crucial, it's when the clay a.k.a. their mind is in their softest form.

Also neuroplasticity holds true for Anxiety Disorder or Depression and almost for every behaviour you have. You have set the mental behavioural pattern, it's just you have to reverse it of which the process is stated in this book.

The mind adapted with the certain feeling of anxiety or thought or memories that gives you depression be it be rational or irrational.

More time you gave to your intrusive thoughts, anxiety or depression, more the wiring was changed which supported the same. And your brain made this your default state. That's why I put emphasis of giving yourself more time to fun lifestyle. More you are busy having fun, more you will slowly change your default state though it will fluctuate in between because you are giving new information to your brain. Plus fun-lifestyle will contribute a lot with the mindsets laid out in the book.

And yeah, if you are critical enough, you have understood by now it is possible to change and reverse mental disorder. At least to a level where you can live your life happily without any irrational worries.

So, just follow the upcoming chapters and the process laid out, and you'll surely achieve your destination.

NOBODY CAN STOP YOU.

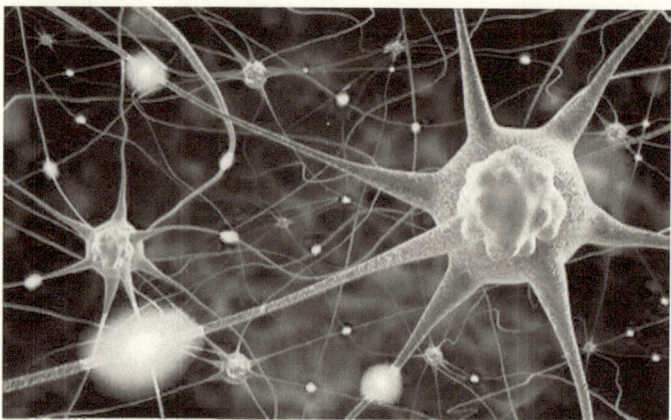

*PICTURE DEPICTING THE NEURON FORMATION IN BRAIN

NEUROPLASTICITY

The Ability of the Brain to Reorganize Itself,
Both in Structure and How It Functions

HOW THE BRAIN CHANGES

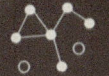 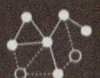 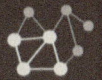

NEUROGENESIS
Continuous generation of new neurons in certain brain regions

NEW SYNAPSES
New skills and experiences create new neural connections

STRENGTHENED SYNAPSES
Repetition and practice strengthens neural connections

WEAKENED SYNAPSES
Connections in the brain that aren't used become weak

NEUROPLASTICITY CAN RESULT FROM:

Traumatic Events · Stress · Social Interaction · Meditation · Emotions

Learning · Paying Attention · Diet · Exercise · New Experiences

CHAPTER 5

OCD IS AN ILLUSION

You think the problem is a particular thought or thinking that's provoking it. It's actually so further away from the truth.

When I had bouts of OCD, from a particular thought, I use to think that particular thought is the cause, later when I had multiple mixed OCD rising from different thoughts or thinking or incidence, I had a huge epiphany.

I realised those thoughts and thinking were just excuses, a medium through which my OCD got provoked, no matter what were the thoughts or themes, the core anxiety and panic I felt was the same. The thought or thinking that I was attaching my OCD to was just a fucking illusion.

I realised it was a mental loop. A loop of negative thought and anxiety which resulted due to years of negative thinking pattern. A loop that makes you feel and think negative. Sometimes it happens due to childhood trauma as well.

Any serious stress, bad lifestyle, negative or unpleasant thinking would have provoked it.

Attaching an OCD to a particular thought or behaviour is very stupid.

And the behaviours that resulted out of having an OCD are just the by-product of the disorder.

If you are behaving awkward cause of OCD. It's okay no need to be harsh on yourself. It's not you that's behaving awkwardly; it's the OCD that's making you sometimes awkward. Accept it heartfully that you behave awkward sometimes, be fine with it, accept it and you would realise that you start to feel better about yourself.

RESISTING CAUSES THE TENSION, ACCEPTING RELEASES THE TENSION.

Also, OCD sometimes makes you think negative about yourself, or make you believe the negative which is all false and illusion. Whenever the negative self-thought comes just remember that it is false and an illusion.

So, all in all, the entire thing we should focus on is the core problem which is the negative mental loop built through years.

The Focus on which is done on this book. So, follow every word.

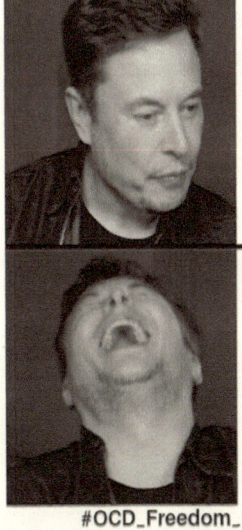

Realising
OCD is an
illusion

Believing
what your
OCD tells
you

#OCD_Freedom_Formula_Book

UNIT 2

MECHANISM OF HEALING

CHAPTER 6

GOD MINDSET

Use **God Mindset** whenever you get overwhelmed by theories or mechanisms, just revert back to this, this has enough power to do the major part of the healing. And another part is discussed in the chapter "**The Formula**". That doesn't mean you ignore the other chapters, every chapter, every section has a role in your healing everything starting from introduction; every section in this book is related.

There is a reason I named it **God Mindset** because I want all of you to follow this mindset like a GOD. Whenever any problem arises recite this mindset. This mindset has immense power if you follow as I directed in this chapter.

Anyways, here goes the "**GOD MINDSET**":

> *"If you (OCD) want to come, come, I don't care"*

The thing is **just let go**, let it do whatever it wants, whatever happens, happens. Even if it is any thought, anxiety, panic attacks, depression, irritation whatever. You don't give a damn now.

Worrying, trying to solve or understand OCD will only increase it.

Best reaction is not to give any reaction.

At beginning it might be a bit difficult but later you will get use to it and will become your automatic response. Imagine someone's trying to tease you, but you don't react, that someone will eventually stop sooner or later.

Whatever thinking comes, let it come, but you won't consciously think or try to solve or control it.

Whatever happens let it happen. It is not a part of you, which you think it is, and that's what gives power to the disorder.

In other words, whatever feeling or thought comes "**let it come, accept it, don't label it good or bad or try to solve and go deep on it.**" Cause the thought itself is irrational and trying to go deep and understand or solve the irrational thought or feeling will only make it worse.

You are not the thought, you are the observer.

So, now the explanation of "you won't consciously think" part:

You won't consciously think:

See, there are two channels of thinking:-

1. Subconscious thinking: thinking that is not in your control, that you don't consciously put effort to think, which comes to huge extent automatically.
2. Conscious thinking: thinking that you do consciously from your side. The one that you are exerting conscious effort.

Now, the 'think' part from the "I won't consciously think" mindset above – I am referring to conscious thinking, not subconscious thinking i.e. the thinking that you do from your side consciously.

Don't try to control the thought that's coming subconsciously, the more you try to stop it, more it will cause the resistance, and more it will irritate. Let it come, accept it, don't label it good or bad.

The problem starts when you try to think about it consciously, which is an old habit that you developed. When you think consciously you give more importance to the particular OCD in your mind.

The common things you think consciously when you have OCD are:

1. Why it's happening to me?
2. God, please help me?
3. How it's happening? (This implies that you are trying to solve it, which is a big No-No.....)
4. It's so irritating...
5. I can't take it
   Etc.......you get the gist
   All these conscious thinking, you will observe whenever you do gives a negative energy to your body, so don't do it.....

But hey, I can't stop the conscious thinking...

No, you are wrong, the thought that comes subconsciously you can't, but the thought that you are going to do consciously you definitely can.

In the beginning, it might seem a bit hard..... With practice, it will become automatic.

So, what you do is

"Whenever the thought comes, recite the **God mindset**, and carry on your work or whatever chores you have"

Just like developing any habit at beginning it seems a bit difficult, but with time you not thinking consciously will turn into a habit and almost your second nature and easy just like learning a guitar or balancing on a bicycle. Any kind of training or learning it takes time but it is with the time that it becomes easier.

Imagine yourself sitting on a platform, and many trains are coming and going.

The trains are like the 'unpleasant feelings and thoughts' they come to the platform, but you don't have to board the train (i.e.: not think about it consciously why and how it has come, and other unnecessary conscious thinking), let it come, and when you don't board the train, it will go eventually. So, it's basically training your mind not to board the train i.e. not to think about it consciously, you know what I mean.

You have inculcated the habit of boarding the train, cut this habit with the process laid out on this chapter and you will be in the path of healing.

Another Bonus mindset:

"*You can only control your mind by not controlling it*", more you try to control, more it will be hard and thus more you become attached to it, the key is in the unattachment and acceptance, if your mind tells you are a loser, or any negative thought you don't have to listen to it, imagine that mind to be a person or anyone who is scolding you; let him/her scold, you don't have to listen to it heart fully and take it to heart. Just don't give a fuck. By the way here by acceptance I don't mean you believe what your mind is telling you, but instead accept that the thought is coming, welcome it but you don't consciously try to go deep on that thought, subconsciously if you are thinking about the thought it is okay.

This subconscious habit of a negative mental loop that you developed happened because at one point you use to do it consciously and now it has become a subconscious habit. Similarly, if you stop going deep on your thought consciously at later point it will too become a subconscious habit and slowly and eventually you break the pattern of the loop.

Another example I can give is suppose you have a nagging friend who teases you on your particular something. The more your friend teases, the more you get irritated. And the more you get irritated, the more your friend enjoys teasing you and as a result your friend teases you more. But if you start loving and accepting the tease, your friend will realise that you are not getting irritated anymore, thus your friend will lose the fun, and eventually stop teasing you. The healing process of your disorder will be very similar to this example.

And again I want to state that the key is in the unattachment and acceptance, not stopping or resisting or controlling it. You should eventually with the process laid out in this book be in such a level that even if it comes, you are not panicking, you be like, okay come, it doesn't matter you are there or not.

*unattachment: not thinking about the thought consciously, if its subconscious than okay.
acceptance: welcome it, being okay with it.

CHAPTER 7

THE FORMULA

So, the **OCD Freedom formula (a.k.a the *2-STEP* healing system)** is as below:

God Mindset + Fun Lifestyle = Process of healing

Fun Lifestyle: Try to get at least for a month a lifestyle where you are free of stress, no work, stay with friends you really connect, if you have no friends still okay, do something that you love and enjoy and have a lot of fun, try to be in an environment or condition that doesn't present extra stress on your brain like studies, project and stuff.

Leave stressing about money, family, and children everything in that month.

Again if a stress is coming sub-consciously due to OCD its okay, but the key is you don't put any extra stress.

Applying all that you have learned till now in this month, you will feel happy to some extent, and see improvement.

Maybe you might hit normal zone, when this happens your brain will get proof and realize you can reach normal zone, this is the point when your wiring will start changing in the positive direction, have a journal or note copy: where you note down the date and proofs of your realizations, this is the point your healing has started.

Now key things to note:

1. When you hit normal zone, you might fear that your OCD might come again anytime, which might be true cause at the beginning normal zone is not that sustainable, with following the process it becomes more permanent later – I have explained thoroughly about this on the chapter "**Fluctuation and Critical points**" with graphs and everything. So, yeah don't be scared that it might come back, it might or it might not, whatever maybe the case be ready, even if it comes don't label it as good or bad, if it comes it comes, if it doesn't then doesn't, don't remain attached to it, accept whatever happens, don't resist and think consciously about it. In addition to it, as I said before don't fear OCD as it doesn't affect anything, you believing that it is a bad thing, makes it something to be feared of, it gets power from that fear and it actually starts effecting.

   It's the fear that affects, not necessarily the OCD itself.

   It's kind of a placebo effect for example if you are feeling little bad or unhealthy, and you keep concentrating on it, telling yourself I am feeling bad, I am feeling sick, you will actually start to feel sick.

   So, just know the rule **OCD doesn't affect anything**, at the beginning be delusional and narcissistic about it, at least it will create some positivity, anything positive is good, later during the process, you will realise by yourself that its fear is a mere illusion.

2. You don't have to do leave for the whole year; a month will be good enough as stated at the beginning of this chapter. Give the brain the proof, and continue with your life. I told you to give a month like this because when there is no stress and you live in a fun

lifestyle, the process works the fastest, plus it will generate a positive proof.

3. Even when you are back to your normal life after that non-stressful month leave. Keep external stress as low as possible. Whenever a negative thought comes keep the **God Mindset** in your mind and recite and go back to the journal which has proofs of the dates when you hit normal zones. (more about this on Chapter-10, **Importance Of Journal**)

CHAPTER 8

HOW TO USE THE OCD FREEDOM FORMULA

First of all let me tell you something, as I said before, all of you who are having access to this book, you all may have different types of OCD, different themes but at the core level the cause is same:

1. A negative thinking pattern in your brain that is set as default.
2. A weak mind that succumbs to the illusion that cannot differentiate between truth and false; illusion and reality.

I see in the groups and forums, clients and OCD sufferers talking about all the external stuff, they try to crack the thoughts or a particular obsessive compulsiveness they have which is the surface layer, that's not necessary, that's not the real problem, that's why I say never try to solve it.

It's like you are a lazy procrastinating person in general and you are searching solution for why can't you wake up in morning and you try beverages like tea/coffee, use alarm clock etc. still you feel sleepy, can't wake up. This is because you are not attacking the real core problem which is in this case that you are a "lazy procrastinating person" which is also a type of a habit, a subconscious loop.

Similarly, in OCD, there might be different thoughts or physical compulsive habits, but you will observe the sensation is same, thus it proves that the problems are not these surface level stuff, it's the core negative mental loop that you have always ignored.

None the less, I am warning, as I have said several times before, **don't discuss or think consciously about these surface layer problems**, never ever. When your mind and belief system becomes strong, you automatically won't think such things.

Your mind is like a muscle, suppose you have weak muscle and try to lift 50 kg barbell bench press, you will probably hurt or fracture yourself, as a result, you won't be able to lift even 10 kg later, that's what you did, first of all you already developed some kind of a habit of irrational thinking or negative thinking consciously, that entered your subconscious mind, which are like bad foods(i.e. irrational thinking) to your brain, which made your mind more weaker to your already weak mind, then when you were in under some kind of stress (like the guy that who tried to lift 50kg), your OCD came to full fruition, and you broke down, depressed (like the guy getting fractured), our mind is like a muscle too.

And imagine the guy who got fractured takes *rest*, gets *good food (diet)*, and now after he got recovered, since genetically he is a weak guy, he next then started with progressive weight training (*Progression*), first with 2.5 kg bench press, after few days his 'muscle memory' got equipped with 2.5 kg weight, then he goes 5 kg and then 10 kg and then 15 kg and eventually step by step he progresses from 15 to ultimately 50 kg or even more than that. It takes little time but it sure is worth it. Now a stress of 50 kg won't affect him anymore.

*Muscle memory: the ability to repeat a specific muscular movement with improved efficiency and accuracy that is acquired through practice and repetition.

Likewise, OCD Freedom Formula is the recovery system for OCD.

First of all, the "*rest*" = 1 month free, that I told you to manage which is possible, do this only after you finished "Understanding the Mechanism" part, that is when you start with "Summarization of the process" from "Application of Mechanism" - where I laid down the process step by step so that you don't get overwhelmed.

Second of all, "*good food (diet)*" = "Fun Lifestyle". Fun decreases OCD and Stress increases OCD. At least at the beginning as your mind is weak. But as you continue with the process fruitfully than with time you will be able to also endure stress and not have OCD, just like how the guy who picked up 50 kg wt at the end did and didn't get fractured.

Third of all is "*Progression*" which we will go deep.

PROGRESSION: In this, you have to use "God Mindset".

The particular compulsive physical habit or ritual you have, stop that and if it is thought or thinking, by now you should know what to do i.e. let it come, don't think about it consciously or try to solve it or anything.

Now, you will have irritation, your mind will try to fuck with you, this is the stage where you have to follow "**God Mindset**" dedicatedly. Your mind will tell not to follow the "God Mindset". This is the first stage and is the most critical stage, once you cross this stage, later stages become comparatively easier (the critical points of different stages is discussed in the chapter "**Fluctuation and Critical Points**")

Now, **if you have a 'fun lifestyle', your conscious mind won't engage in the thought so much, it will get diverted and following the "God Mindset" becomes easier.**

Now, the particular obsessive thought or physical compulsive habit that you believed so much consciously, you will realize after passing through that first stage that it was false, and you will realize the particular surface layer thing that caused your irritation, it doesn't have any effect.

And this is where your healing process starts, but since its beginning, you might again get the thought and irritation again, but it will lose its power it had gradually with time, healing process will be similar to that of man in the village (refer: chapter "**Belief System and how it works**"), where at the end you will get enough prove and positivity that your OCD won't have any power any more. Use the same process for any kind of irrational thought or physical compulsive habit, and slowly you will realize the truth and your mind will be able to comprehend the truth from the illusion slowly.

*In between your starting critical stage and healed stage, you will pass through few fluctuating stages.

CHAPTER 9

HOW OCD FREEDOM FORMULA WILL WORK

Let me give you a muscle building analogy:

Suppose you are trying to do pull up with your whole bodyweight, it will be difficult at the beginning.

So, you start part by part, little by little which are called progressions. With time you'll be able to do 1, but that doing of 1 pull up you had to give a lot of effort, maybe months or days.

But as time goes, with consistent workout and with proper diet your muscle strength builds, then even that 1 pull up becomes easier, after few days of workout even 2nd pull up becomes easy, then 3rd, 4th.......eventually even 10th pull up becomes easier and possible at the end.

It takes time but sure it's worth it.

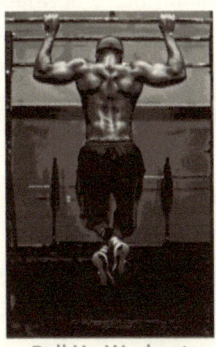

Pull Up Workout

Later, even bodyweight pull up as a whole becomes easy for you, and you can add extra weight for pull up.

Because once you can do pull up, you can always do pull up, brain gets prove and registers it, kind of like muscle memory, similar case when you first balance in a bicycle you give your brain proof that you can do it and eventually you learn riding bicycle, which becomes almost subconscious for you later and you don't have to think, and you can just ride bicycle smooth as butter.

That's why I said to keep journal or note copy, where you can note down the day you have been happy or been in the normal zone so that you give proof to your brain that you can achieve normal zone or be happy even if you have OCD.

So, you can revert back to it whenever you feel down or succumb to the negative illusion your OCD is trying to feed you, which is bullshit.

Same way, likewise for your mind:

Following the "**God mindset**" is the exercise and diet is the "**fun-lifestyle**" where you have least external stress and more fun as possible. In fun-lifestyle stress tends to be less and one is less likely to think consciously which in turn contributes to the working of the god-mindset and thus the healing process becomes faster and easier.

As time passes, you will hit more normal zones, your brain will get more proofs how stupid OCD is, and thus your mind becomes stronger, and less affected you get.

There will be little fluctuations between normal zone and OCD zone but with time, following the process dedicatedly and consistently you will eventually get healed.

CHAPTER 10

IMPORTANCE OF JOURNAL

Journal or Notebook helps to keep track of the proofs such as you can be happy even with OCD or your realization that it(OCD) is bullshit etc.

How it helps:- Suppose you experience a day where you have been happy or experienced a normal zone, note it down: the positive experiences along with the date; by doing these, you are giving new information to your brain, which helps to change the wiring of your brain on a deep subconscious level, plus it produces a reference proof, since it's hard to sustain normal zone at beginning, when you fall back to OCD or when your mind is feeding you with bullshit irrational false negative thoughts, you can refer back to the journal which has the actual proof of your realization and be aware at the moment that whatever your mind is feeding you is bullshit and thus helps you to stay unattached to it, and thus helping you not to part in it consciously.

Plus it builds data of proofs that will contradict your present false beliefs and knowledge about OCD. Thus, it helps to build an understanding of the disorder and even yourself which gives you an extra edge.

Let me give you an example: Suppose you have an OCD of arranging books or any ritual, and now you following OCD Freedom Formula, and you are not doing that particular ritual, your mind will tell you something bad will happen (will be explained more in **Fluctuation and Critical points** chapter), whatever it may be, you follow the **OCD Freedom Formula** strictly, let the thoughts come, you don't care or think consciously about it, instead you accept it, your OCD might go higher temporarily, given that you are having a fun lifestyle, after a point it will actually become lower with relatively lesser affect than initial stage.

Like a hill, it goes to peak, after that it drops. After some time you might achieve a normal zone.

Now, you note it in a journal your surpassing of the fear, you note the date when you hit the normal zone, you realise all the fear you had was irrational, you know now how it makes the fear seem so real but it's so fake, how it makes your power of understanding so weak that you start believing irrational stuff.

Date	Realizations
17/03/2013	Today first time reached normal zone. That means its possible to reach it. Probably, it is the beginning phase, that's why it might not be consistent. But following the process it definitely will become. Also reaching the normal zone, I realized the fact that OCD use to tell me, I can't reach normal zone was a Lie. That probably means everything it tells is a big fat lie.

The picture depicted is the example of how you make your Journal. Its very simple, just two columns, with headings "Date" and "Realizations".

Now, when you write realizations in a journal, you give new information to your brain, and that rewires your false beliefs, knowledge, fear and thus your mind becomes stronger subconsciously even if it is 1%. These small one percents add up and heals you in the long run.

So, again when you get OCD, you revert back to the journal to look back at the truth, which will give you strength to deal with the false belief during OCD zone.

In addition to this, when you look at it during your 'rebound OCD times' or 'fluctuation times', it cheers and motivates you up.

Note: There will be fluctuation, you will be in OCD, then normal, then OCD, again normal, and so on but with each time you achieve normal zone, your brain gets more proof of OCD being false and bullshit, a mere illusion and eventually you achieve consistent normal zone and thus get healed. The further explanation on this is done on the chapter "**Fluctuation and Critical points**".

CHAPTER 11

BELIEF SYSTEM

Let me give you an analogy:

Imagine you are living in a village and there is a small mountain in your village and every villager says nobody can climb it, it's impossible, everyone has believed and accepted the idea of not able to climb the mountain, and thus it has become a self-fulfilling prophecy for everyone.

An average person's belief system in that village at that point will be like Nah, it's pretty damn difficult and dangerous and impossible to climb the mountain, and there is fear in everybody's mind including yours which is false and illusion, which was created due to believing the illusion in the first place.

Now the key point here is, imagine those villagers to be your 'Negative thinking' that keeps on stating that, no you can't do it, your life is fucked, no hope, makes you feel like it's impossible etc. which is not true, because it's an illusion, you just believing the illusion gives it power and nothing else.

OCD is same.

Okay now let's continue the story, after some days you hear a man climbed the mountain, he gets an appraisal by the village. And at this point your fear decreases consciously or subconsciously, even if it is 1%, you start to think maybe it's possible, your negative thinking and fear decreases to some extent, your brain gets a proof of a possibility, a hope. But still a majority of villagers stating that he got lucky. Even if you are believing the majority, but still the fact is that your brain got a little proof that it is possible. (But a better thing here would be to believe the positive information - that it's possible even if it is small.)

Similarly, when you realize the first time that you can be happy with OCD or reach the normal zone first time and you write down the realization in a journal(writing down helps to imprint the information better by the brain consciously), you give information to your brain that you can reach normal zone(just like how you became little positive when you heard that a man climbed the mountain for the first time from the village, which gave information to your brain that its possible to climb the mountain). This gives a sense of positivity and hope, and as I said before it might be fluctuating from positive to negative to positive and so on, since you had years of negative thinking, the trauma will be strong at beginning but with time the more you hit the normal zone and happy state, more your brain gets the new information consciously and subconsciously and more your brain becomes positive, and to be honest you reach a point, even when you have compulsive thinking it doesn't even affect you, cause now you are in a position, you know deep down consciously and subconsciously that it's bullshit .

So, where was I, yeah after you heard that the man climbed the mountain you got a slight touch of positivity. After a few days, you hear a woman climbed the mountain, now your fear decreases more, hence more hope, but still, there are villagers much lesser compared to before though, who are still preaching the negativity of it not being possible, but your brain has got more proofs now.

Later, you found out even some children climbed the mountain, now your fear has decreased more and to a huge extent and now your inner willpower is starting to increase, as your brain is getting more proof that its possible but still there are few negative people (but decreased to much extent compared to previous), and majority villagers now becoming positive about it. (i.e. in terms of OCD when you hit more normal zone, you start becoming more positive about it and the fear decreases drastically.)

And finally at the end, you find several groups of people climbing the mountain (in terms of OCD your positivity has become more) and you realize it was easy and you realize it was just an illusion of fear after all, that the negative people imposed on the villagers, you realize without the fear, the task of climbing the mountain, is not that hard, at this point now, you don't care the slight comments of remaining negative people and their pessimistic talk.

And finally you too climb the mountain, there might be a slight tinch of fear but you make it.

Similar manner is how you get healed from OCD. You reach the normal zone so much, clear so many illusions e.g.: related to religious OCD, POCD, HOCD, certain thought OCD etc. that you realize its tricks and it has no power left and eventually with time you get healed. And your fear is never the same.

Another example of the power of Belief System from a real-life incident:

Up until 1954, it was a mainstream thought amongst essentially any professional athlete that running a mile (1.6kms) in under 4 minutes was simply not possible.

The human body simply couldn't physically sustain such pace without collapsing under pressure.

For years, runners had been striving against the clock, but the elusive 4 minutes had always beaten them.

Like an unconquerable mountain, the closer it was approached, the more daunting it seemed.

This was truly the holy grail of athletic achievement.

The four-minute mile stood for decades - and every single expert involved predicted that if anyone were to ever break it, it must happen under a very specific set of circumstances: Perfect weather - 20 degrees and no wind to be exact; on a particular type of track - hard, dry clay. And in front of a huge crowd urging the runner on to his best ever performance.

Essentially, there would need to be a lot of 'luck' involved.

...Yet Roger Bannister did it on a cold day, on a wet track, at a small meet in Oxford, before a relatively small crowd.

And it was anything but 'luck'.

When he did so, even his most bitter rivals breathed a sigh of relief.

'At last, somebody fucking did it!'

Any guesses as to what happened after Bannister shattered everyone's belief that "running a mile in under 4 minutes was not possible?"

Yep,

Every motherfucker and his dog started running a mile in under four minutes.

And it wasn't because their conditioning, pace or stamina suddenly improved.

It was because Bannister had liberated them from their self-imposed mental prison.

The barrier was much more of a psychological one than a physical one.

'Human beings act in alignment with what they perceive to be as true about themselves and the environment in which they operate in'.

If you truly understand it, it will change your life.

Your belief systems (subconscious mind), LITERALLY HAS THE FUCKING ABILITY TO ALTER BEHAVIOURAL FUNCTIONS IN YOUR PHYSICAL BODY.

If you believe that you're only entitled to your thoughts, that's all you'll get, but if you think you are independent of your thoughts (i.e. your thoughts doesn't affect you) and you can be happy irrespective of it, you will receive all the happiness and positivity that is there.

-> Your subconscious brain will then allow you to freely be the fucking man around the low hanging fruit, and shut down the negativity.

One more thing I want to tell you about belief system is that your I.Q, face, body, height, hair etc. can or might be genetic. But remember...

Belief System is never genetic.

It's something you develop on your own.

Anybody can develop their belief system. Nobody is born with more or less belief system than others.

And for you, I already laid out how you would develop your belief system in terms of OCD. It's a process after all, anybody can develop it. So, follow the process laid out in this book with utmost sincerity.

No excuse.

CHAPTER 12

FLUCTUATION AND CRITICAL POINTS

As mentioned in the chapter "**How to use OCD Freedom Formula**", the first stage will be the most critical.

You will go through a stage temporarily which will be a little difficult than your present stage, but with following the process, you will realize even though OCD is there it doesn't affect you that much, following the process laid out in the chapter "**How to use OCD Freedom Formula**" you might reach normal zone, and as I said there will be fluctuation like you will reach normal zone, then again OCD zone, key thing here is : when you first reach normal zone you will have subconscious fear like OH! Please OCD don't come again, don't do that - be okay even if OCD comes again, accept it, don't think about it consciously, don't label it good or bad, don't try to solve why it has come again, and shit like that. Just follow the process.

Following the process, what will happen is, you will observe that you will be in the normal zone, and after sometime get OCD again(even if you get OCD, keep on following the process, trust the process no matter what, and I promise, you will witness light at the end of the tunnel) than again you will be in the normal zone, again OCD, again normal zone, this will continue, but the key thing is each time you hit normal zone, your brain gets the information that it is possible to be in normal zone even with OCD, hence adding positivity with each hit of normal zone, and with time you will ultimately reach a point where your normal zone will be more consistent. Your past trauma may haunt you at times (depending on the person) but it won't have any power now because your brain has got enough proof. And at this point you are a healed person.

Again remember: The beginning is the most critical part, your mind might try to trick you not to follow the process, at that point you must trust the process, trust this program like a GOD.

Later, it becomes much easier for you to follow the process because at the beginning you are negative; you feel it's impossible to come out because you are in an illusion, just like that person who thought he couldn't climb the mountain cause of the negative illusion put forward by his villagers. Trusting the process you will recognize the illusion and get out of it.

At beginning don't talk about or discuss your OCD with anyone just follow the process laid out in this book, cause more you discuss negative stuff(OCD), more you are reminding your brain of it subconsciously.

*Following there are the graphs of different phases and stages: your progression from initial OCD zone to consistent normal zone to healed stage.

Below is the graph of the first critical stage:

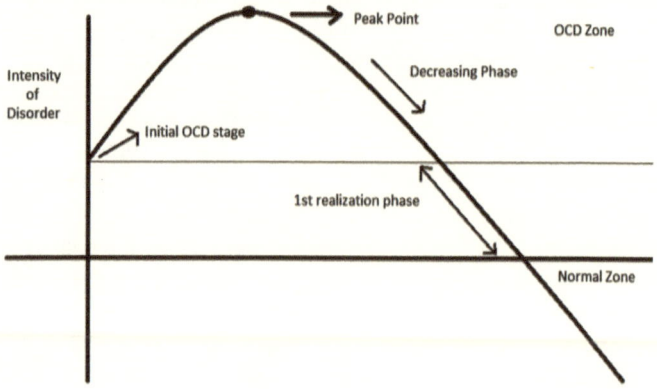

Now, after the hitting of peak point, there will be this decreasing phase, there might be again increasing phase (will differ with respect to the person), "don't panic here", it's normal, again I say don't panic accept it as I said before, more you accept it, lesser will be its effects. After decreasing phase, you will achieve an OCD stage much lesser than your 'Initial OCD stage', that is when you achieve your 1st realization and further continuing the process you will definitely achieve normal zone.

As I said, there will be multiple decreasing and increasing 'OCD phases', depending on the trauma that OCD left with you.

Nothing to worry, I probably had one of the worst OCD, multiple mixed OCD. Literally thousands of multiple thoughts at once. If me following the process can get healed than anybody can get healed.

So, as I was saying there will be a roller coaster of increasing and decreasing phases, and eventually you will hit the normal zone, again OCD zone and so on which is natural at beginning and yeah remember "you can be happy in OCD too".

So, the basic graph of the fluctuation will be as follows, keep in mind the no. of loops might differ with respect to people.

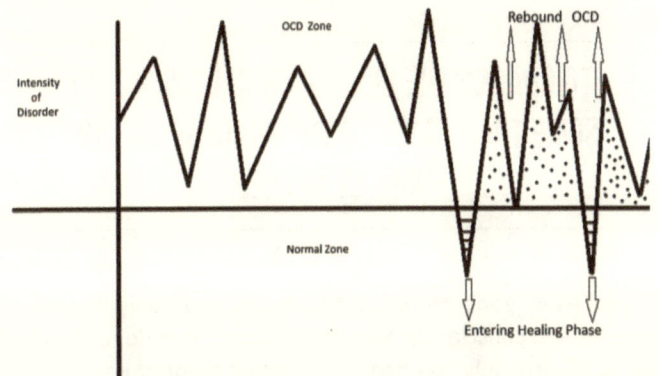

➢ **"Entering Healing Phase"**: This is the phase your brain records that it's possible to get healed from OCD and your brain starts recognizing illusion (write in journal or note copy to imprint the information better in form of 'dates and realization').

The more you reach this zone, the more your brain get proofs, the more your brain registers it, the more you come out of the illusion.

➢ **"Rebound OCD"**: These are negative thoughts and fear from your past OCD trauma, once you hit the normal zone, you might again get back to OCD zone or at peak level (very less likely), and again I say: don't panic here, accept it even if it comes, even when you reach normal zone, don't have the fear that your OCD will come again or not. Be ready, even if it comes. It might come again because your 'mind muscle-your belief system' is not strong yet at beginning and also the experience of normal zones might be very less at beginning which is obvious since you are only starting out the process.

And keep in mind that the years and months of OCD has changed the wiring of your brain (the process of your brain which is known as neuroplasticity).

TO CHANGE THE WIRING AGAIN IT WILL TAKE SOME TIME. STICK TO THE PROCESS AND YOU WILL BE HEALED.

If you have gone from normal to OCD, it only happened because you consciously or subconsciously were doing negative thoughts, probably you had stress at that point of your life and boom with time you changed the wiring of your brain and started to have OCD.

Whatever OCD you have, with various habits, thinking or feeling but the core reason is you have weak mind muscle or weak belief system , that helped in the formation of the negative wiring in your brain with negative mental loops that gives you unpleasant feelings and thoughts. And going too deep to the thoughts is similar to like you having a weak body and trying to lift 50 kg wt(similar to huge stress or overthinking) with you having weak strength(similar to feeble mind in case of OCD).

The bottom-line is if you can go from normal to OCD, you can definitely return from OCD to normal.

Again, when you are in normal zone at beginning, since you are just starting out, your negative side of mind is still little strong (depending on the person) don't try to block the negative thoughts, let it come, but you don't think about it consciously, you thinking about it consciously might make it increase again.

Now, the basic gist is you will hit multiple loops of increasing phase, decreasing phase, and normal zone.

With time, in the loop, the peak point will decrease, and normal zone will increase and after some more time, you will reach a point where there are almost no loops you have consistent normal zone. In this consistent zone, your past trauma might haunt you at times which I call "**minor temporary fluctuation**" (again depends on the person and even it happens don't panic, it won't affect as before, just recite the **God Mindset**) it won't have any power as before cause your brain now has got enough proof. At this point, you are almost a healed person. Further continuing the process you will be in healed stage.

The overall graph showing the progression of how you get healed is as follows:

OCD FREEDOM FORMULA

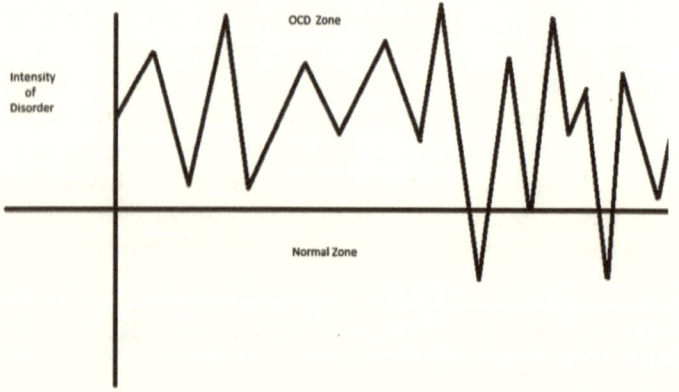

*when you just start to hit normal zone

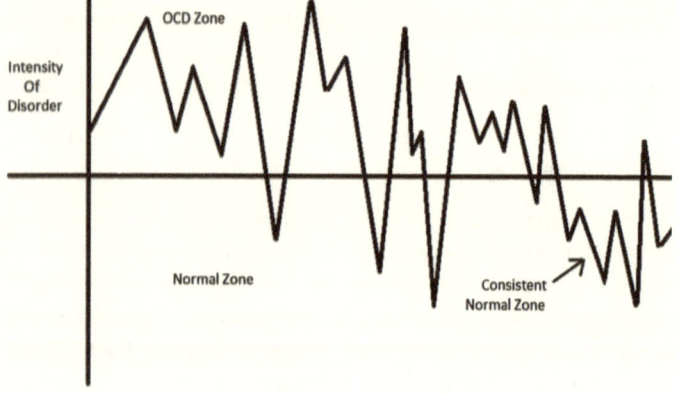

*As you start to hit more normal zones, it slowly becomes more consistent and less fluctuating

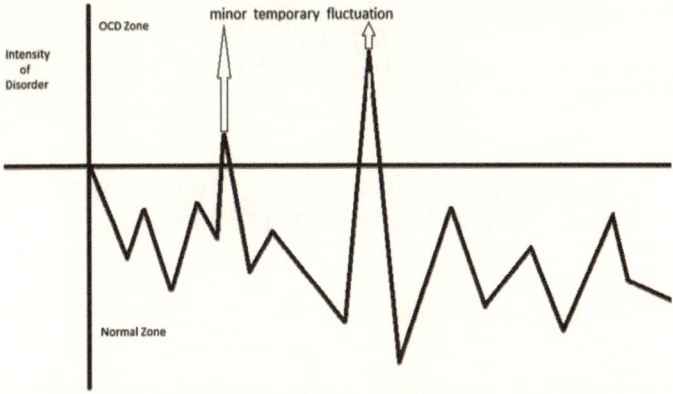

*in between your 'consistent normal zone' there might be 'minor temporary fluctuation' at times which doesn't last long at all and plus its effect will be really low compared to your previous OCD stage and even if it comes welcome it, accept it and follow the God Mindset. As you progress further you won't even be needing a fun lifestyle, God Mindset becomes enough.

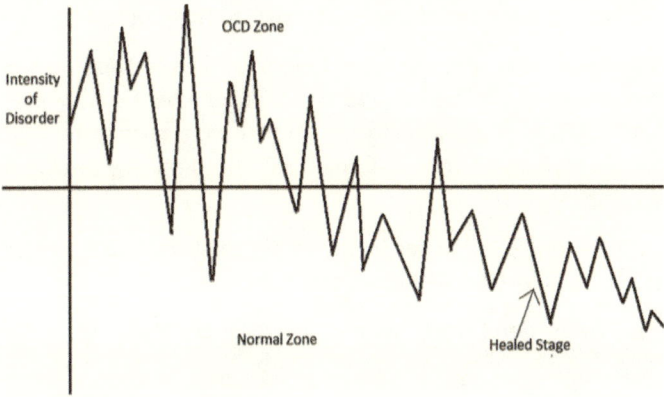

*the overall process from your 'initial stage' to 'Healed stage'. And yeah as I said before the fluctuation will differ with respect to the person but the process will be same.

CHAPTER 13

STICKING TO MINDSETS

This is a very small chapter only to remind you of the importance of the mindsets both the core mindsets and '**GOD Mindset**'.

Stick to the mindsets no matter what.

Your brain will try to trick you, make you not to continue the process, make you feel like it's okay to think consciously.

Again, I am saying no matter what, stick to the process.

Take the help of a Journal or notebook where you keep track or remember the reference you had that you were happy even with OCD, it is possible to hit Normal zone even with OCD. Always remember that your mind will try to make you believe something else.

Your mind will try to get to you in old thinking, but if you are using "fun lifestyle" diet it can't so much.

By the way, don't worry; it only happens in the initial stage little bit.

After a few days or months, you will get the hold of it. And slowly it will become second nature.

*core mindsets: Mindsets mentioned in this book other than the God Mindset. If you want to get all the core mindsets in one chapter go to "Core Mindsets" from Unit-4: Summarization of the process, plus you have some bonus core mindsets there.

CHAPTER 14

POWER OF ACCEPTANCE

Acceptance is a key part of the process laid out in this book and has been mentioned many times on various chapters. I don't want you to miss out on this. So, I had to make a chapter on this to go a little in-depth.

By the way here by acceptance I don't mean you believe what your mind is telling you, but instead accept that the thought is coming, welcome it but you don't consciously try to go deep on that thought, subconsciously if you are thinking about the thought it is okay.

Acceptance of the thought not what the thought is telling you.

Acceptance is so powerful that when it is done right, you can be happy in any condition, and if it's really serious condition at least you won't panic.

Acceptance decreases stress, decreases insecurity, decreases any other burden, keeps you present and calm.

When you are having OCD, try resisting it for a while.

How do you feel?

You feel an irritation right.

And then try accepting it.

You will realize, it feels much better as compared to resisting it.

Just as with time if you keep on resisting OCD, it keeps on increasing.

Similarly, just as with time if you accept OCD, it decreases, especially the irritation feeling.

Accept that OCD is there with you, it doesn't matter anymore, if it comes or goes or when it comes or goes doesn't matter to you.

If you truly accept OCD, you wouldn't mind whether it is there with you all day or not.

When it comes you won't even react to it or resist it. Cause you have truly accepted it.

It's like a guest to you.

ACCEPT OCD AND REMAIN UNATTACHED TO IT.

And when I say **"remain unattached to it"** I mean don't take part in the OCD consciously as I mentioned before.

If it is happening in the background subconsciously let it happen.

Let the guest come, do whatever it wants. Accept the guest but no need to deal with him.

CHAPTER 15

THOUGHT JUMPS

If like me you had multiple mixed OCD, you will have thought-jumps.

From one thing or topic to another, back to back to back sometimes.

As I stated before your mind is weak now.

In fracture mode.

Never be like 'why is it happening with me', 'Oh no! I can't take it' and stuff like that...

Thoughts on which your mind jumps are external.

It is just that your mind cannot assess what's rational and what's irrational.

If you follow the process dedicatedly and consistently, your mind will slowly become strong and identify those irrational thoughts.

Following the process, you will be hitting more normal zones from time to time. Of course, the normal zones won't be continuous, there will be fluctuation little bit.

Your mind will become stronger as your brain gets more proofs. You have no idea how much mind is similar to muscle.

Anybody who goes to the gym or any fitness stuff, and doing his fitness naturally, he doesn't get big automatically next day, with time and progressions, they eventually get big and lift off more weights. Sometimes in the fitness process, they hit a plateau (can't lift more weight or don't get big), after sometime or some days they break the plateau and lift more i.e. they too have fluctuation but eventually with following the process for getting fit, they too get stronger and bigger.

ALL YOU NEED IS PATIENCE, DEDICATION AND CONSISTENCY.

If you have these three qualities.

Nobody can stop you.

You will be healed to the level you can live your daily life happily at the very least.

And yeah...

Those "**Thought Jumps**" should give you a huge realization like it gave to me i.e. in spite of so many external thought jumps, the core anxiety is same(yeah some anxiety may have more effect and some less irrespective of that anxiety will be there).

That should give you an on-hand epiphany that those external thoughts are an illusion, a mere medium.

You would feel anxiety anyway; your mind is just finding an excuse in disguise of a thought or compulsive behaviour.

This should make you further realize that how much time you are wasting, thinking or discussing or trying to solve those external thoughts or should I say external excuse/ illusion/medium.

If not this thought than other.

So, stop focussing on the thought consciously.

I see in forums and groups people discussing their external thought problem, trying to solve it which further makes their OCD stronger sub-consciously.

If you are trying to solve or discuss irrational stuff consciously, your mind will obviously give you irrational results.

Bottom-line is don't try to think about your thoughts consciously, that's it. It's actually simple though it seems hard. As I said before, with any habit it will seem a bit hard at the beginning but with time it will become automatic just like riding a bicycle.

Whenever those thought comes just recite the "**GOD Mindset**" and continue with the process.

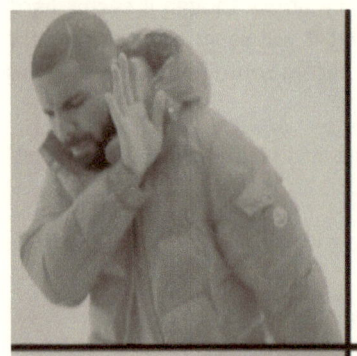

Resisting
OCD

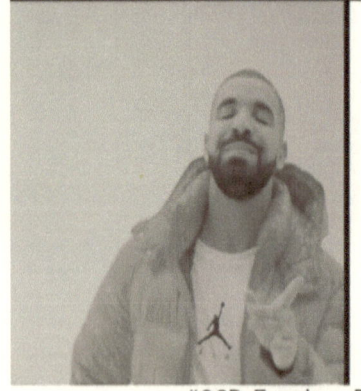

Accepting
OCD

#OCD_Freedom_Formula_Book

UNIT 3

MECHANISM OF SELF-SABOTAGING

CHAPTER 16

HEALING BLOCKERS

There are some habits that you have developed, consciously or unconsciously that directly or indirectly trained your mind to believe in irrational stuff, this surely happened especially from childhood.

I am sure, I will be crushing some of your beliefs in this section, but it is for your own good if you follow, you will heal fast if you ignore you are just being an obstacle to yourself.

These bad habits that you might have developed from childhood needs to be stopped. Don't just force and try to remove these habits, do it steady and slow.

These bad habits have contributed to the weakening of your Belief System.

I will go straight forward and point it out below:

1. **Superstitious Belief**: Having superstitious beliefs gives your mind an outdoor to believe in irrational stuff (just like bad food in your diet). A bad negative habit and programming that you gave to your mind. You are literally training your mind to believe in irrational stuff. This habit feeds OCD. If you have superstitious belief try to set away from it, little by little.

2. **Desperate Praying**: By doing it you are subconsciously telling your mind, that you are weak, you have no other way, it takes you to a negative spiral, stops you

to think constructively. Weakens your belief system, the moment you do desperate praying you give signal to your brain that you are helpless and weak, which further weakens your belief system, crushes positive belief, lose hope etc. You subconsciously signal your brain that you are helpless and miserable and you actually start to feel that way.

Instead, whenever you are in a trouble, you should believe in yourself, try to find a solution, in that way you train your mind to develop self-belief and self-trust. Thus, you give more power to yourself instead of depending on an external source. And, thus strengthen your belief system.

Don't mistake hoping and praying as same.

Desperate Praying is basically crying for help in a begging way which gives a negative signal to your brain.

While hope is a positive thought someday something good might happen. This gives a positive vibe to you, your body, mind and soul.

3. **Don't believe in gemstone, zodiac signs and other external shit:** One person that you should have a belief is in yourself. Self- belief is the best. More than gemstone or zodiac or even GOD.

It's you. You come first.

Believe in yourself more than anything.

All the three points I stated above if you cultivate will instil a positive mental habit. Self-trust will increase. You will depend more on yourself.

And thus strengthen more of your belief system.

CHAPTER 17

OCD AND RELATIONSHIP

When I say relationship, it can be anything, a relationship with your spouse, boyfriend/girlfriend, parents, friends etc.

It is necessary that you don't take too stress on a relationship.

Sometimes, a small thing or issue can make you pissed off, sad or upset. Since you are in OCD never take the small stuff seriously i.e.: **you don't think about it consciously if you are stressing subconsciously but not consciously taking part on it than nothing major would happen**. Again, just like any habit at the beginning, it will be a bit difficult, but with time, it becomes a part of you. And by not taking part in it consciously I mean, don't go deep on those issues consciously, subconsciously let it happen whatever happens.

If you were in a normal zone, probably it wouldn't be the same case; you would be chill about this small stuff.

Technically, in a relationship even if it is with your friends, society, don't feel or take deeply if they are hard on you, ignore you or whatever at times if it happens.

Remember this, it even applies to general people, don't care if someone hates, talks bad at you, what you should care is about your particular purpose at a particular time.

Importance Of purpose: Your purpose might be hitting the next target at your job, dancing, singing, sports...Getting in shape whatever. What purpose does is, it helps you to cut all the noise such as what people are saying to you, think about you and helps you realise what bullshit and petty this habit of caring about people is.

*You can know your purpose or passion by following the chapter "**Finding your Passion**" from Unit-4

The "Life is an adventure" mindset to cut all the other people issue, upset over petty stuff & noises:

"Everything is temporary, as time goes, what people say or think, things happened regarding your relationship everything, everyone will go, everything is so temporary, why are you crying, why are you stressing about it, everything is temporary, why are you stressing about temporary stuff, your girlfriend/boyfriend dumped you. You still have so many years, it's just a part of a few beginning chapters of your life, there are so many chapters left, why are you crying over the first few chapters, and even if it is from the later chapters, there are still many parts left, story has not ended yet, anything bad happened or that might in your life is temporary, life itself is temporary, take life as an adventure, even bad times are fun and even good times are fun, remain unattached to the things that produces negativity in your life and stop stressing consciously over things that make you negative(if it is subconscious, that's okay it will come and go). Life is too short for that, follow your dreams, do what you love, go to a party, club, dance, sing and don't give a fuck."

Whenever you see yourself crying over any petty stuff - friends, family, society, gf/bf...I mean like anything, read the above mindset, it will make you grounded, present and focused.

Key thing here:

The mindsets – "**God mindset**" and "**Life is an adventure**": note it in the phone or copy or whatever, so that you can look at any time when you need.

Internalising this mindset will keep you at peace and nothing can stop you to be happy.

Add a "fun lifestyle" which will act as a steroid.

*INTERNALISING OR INTERNALISATION: value or beliefs or behaviour that becomes subconscious and automatic through consistent application.

Follow the mindsets and the process, have fun, do your daily activity. Don't think or talk about OCD as possible, I already stated in the "**OCD Paradox**" chapter 19, why that is.

In case OCD is affecting your important work, say this to yourself *"If you (subconscious OCD thought) come, come, I don't care, I will do my work, shits (works) got to be done than shits (works) got to be done* (or your own version of it)" and continue with your work – this really works in terms of important tasks or work. Because it gives a flight or fight response. Like, suppose you are a lazy person can't run that fast, but if suddenly there is a hungry tiger behind you, you will forget your idea of being lazy completely and you will actually run so fast that you never thought of; you probably got now a gist of what I meant by flight or fight response.

When it comes to being social, you might get pissed off at small stuff, hold it there remember "**life is an adventure**" mindset. And drop your ego since you are still in a healing phase.

CHAPTER 18

TABOO THOUGHTS

It's an issue that many people having OCD have told they faced.

Whether it is illegal sexual thoughts, or incest or whatever.

The fact of the matter is, you feel like you are guilty to have that thought.

You try to resist it, and more you resist, more you go deep into those thoughts.

I guarantee every single person had a taboo thought cross their mind even it is for a split second.

The only difference is since most of the people are normal, they can quickly assess that what they are thinking is wrong, and immediately remove that thinking from their head.

Since you are suffering from OCD, your mind gets hold of that thought and gets obsessed with it. For you the best thing would be not to take part in the thought consciously, because more you would take part in the thought consciously more you would go deep.

Plus, if possible change the environment if it's supporting the creation of the thought.

Also, loneliness would definitely contribute in these thoughts.

So, try being busy with something.

Something you are passionate about, it will let you open.

In addition, since you are passionate about that particular thing of yours, you won't even get bored.

And ya again I say don't feel guilty, its not your fault.

You just have an unstable mind.

With time and following the process it will become okay.

CHAPTER 19

OCD PARADOX

One of the paradoxes is already stated to you in the previous chapter i.e.: **the more you resist or fight OCD, the more it will create problem.**

The more you accept and be okay and happy with OCD the lesser becomes its intensity.

And yeah another key paradox that I am going to explain is:

"*Don't put a time when you will get healed, more you do that, more there is a chance of making the process uneasy*":

Suppose you put a time like example after 3 months or 6 months, you will become healed, you will be all the time thinking about OCD as a result (which is opposite of what you are trying to do).

Putting expectations are vague, because the real-time might differ according to the person, so don't put expectations, you will get heal no doubt, but putting expectations will make you impatient, will create stress and stress supports OCD which we don't want.

The paradox is "**Not to think about OCD consciously as much as possible and follow the process.**" (As with any habit it might be difficult at the beginning but with time it will be automatic)

Don't think about OCD; only think about happy and positive stuff as possible.

So, the trick here is to think like OCD is a part of your life now, you are happy even if you get little relief from where you were initially, and follow the process laid out in this program.

This will keep you happy and content.

One thing about happiness you should know that it's relative: if a poor guy gets a loaf of bread he will be happy all day, but if a middle class or rich person gets the same probably nothing compared to the poor guy. Expectation decreases the relativeness.

'IT'S BETTER TO BE SURPRISED THAN TO EXPECT'.

For example, you had an exam you thought you will fail but instead, you somehow pass, that will give you more happiness than if you expected 95% and you ended up getting 80%.

So, if you keep no expectations, even with little improvement you will be happy, which in turn will give you more boost and happiness, which will decrease pain, fear, stress at a more powerful rate.

If you have OCD, don't discuss about your OCD with your friends, family and acquaintances, or even if you are a part of a group, don't discuss problems, don't share sadness, only talk about happy stuff, fun stuff, the emotion of fun and happiness that is what you should surround yourself with.

The more you talk about OCD and problem, more subconsciously you are giving the signal to your brain that you are helpless and weak and reminding your brain of it. Have you ever felt when you share problems in a group, you start to accept that you are helpless, kind of hopelessness seems to surround you more, you feel that negative energy that makes you weak. You get a temporary relief when somebody responses to your issue but after sometime again back to the same zone. Don't misconstrue what I said to not share your issue when necessary with a professional or a person who really understands it. But in general don't talk or discuss about it, reminding your brain of it, just share and discuss happy stuff as much as possible.

Talk and discuss and share happy stuff, in the beginning, you might have to give a little push, later like any habit it becomes automatic and tell yourself even if I have OCD I am all right, it doesn't have any effect.

The key here is you don't consciously try to remind your brain of OCD. Live your life in such a way that you don't have to consciously think or talk about OCD as much as possible.

And **fun-lifestyle** helps you to do this the best.

"Keep your requirements for happiness as low as possible "

If you can eat and sleep and have a hobby or something to have fun that should be enough to make you happy. If you can't sleep or eat follow **OCD Freedom Formula** that will do the work. And do something fun like : going to cinemas with friends to hang out, or alone doesn't matter; do something you love : music, art, science whatever, or go to a party, go out of your comfort zone and dance your full(this works the best by the way) and don't give a fuck.

So, only fun, no thinking consciously or talking about OCD, use the **God mindset** when it is severe, otherwise fun lifestyle is enough. And when you hit normal zone write and note it in your journal on your happy days.

*Two sentences or something similar that I have repeated many times:

1. Don't think consciously about it, if it's subconscious than okay.

2. At beginning it will be a bit hard, later it will become automatic.

This is because I know your brain would try to make you not follow it, make excuses, try to make you believe the opposite or stop you to do the correct thing.

See, I want you to heal.

And for that if I have to repeat a certain thing on and on to hammer it into your brain.

I will gladly do it.

CHAPTER 20

HOW TO GET CONTROL OVER YOUR SUICIDAL THOUGHTS

First let me explain why do you develop a suicidal thought in the first place.

See, suicidal thought is basically a build up of your fear and conscious thinking on your OCD.

As I said before you have two channels of thinking:

One being "**conscious**".

And other being "**subconscious**".

In addition to it you were constantly reminding your brain of your OCD by following ways:

1. Negative self-talking consciously about it.
    For example: I can't take it anymore, it's killing me, this feels so hopeless etc. etc.
    When you do such negative self-talk, you are giving negative message to your brain.
    Whatever you tell your brain, it will just accept, it doesn't filter.
    If the self-talking is happening sub-consciously let it happen.
    No need to worry about subconscious self-talking.
    That's not you, that's OCD.

Don't get attached to it.

At least don't do self-talking consciously.

Instead let it happen whatever happens, and you don't consciously think or talk about it or try to solve it.

2. By sharing or discussing your misery, how OCD has made your life pathetic, and stuff like that.

Don't do it.

If you had to share with a professional that's a different case.

But if you are doing as in general and quite often, than don't.

Otherwise if you are sharing or discussing such stuff, your brain will turn it more into reality because you are giving negative message to your brain and constantly consciously reminding your brain of it.

Instead what you do is start to accept OCD.

Practice gratitude; be happy with small small things in your life no matter how small it is.

Just imagine when you first had OCD, if you just focussed on the positive side and not thinking about it consciously, instead of focussing on how it's making you feel anxious, going deep on it and trying to solve it, you would be in a better condition right now.

Cause at the very first beginning your OCD was probably mild.

But you grew its power by doing and developing all the wrong ways of dealing with it and forming it into a habit.

And thus your OCD became stronger and severe.

And in this book I am giving all the habits and mindsets that will reverse it.

And yeah...

Don't fight OCD, accept OCD.

Like really do it.

You just start accepting it whenever it comes.

Don't label it good or bad. Just don't.

In OCD world, Fear is opposite of Acceptance.
If fearing OCD increases its power.
Then, definitely accepting OCD will decrease its power.
Point Blank Period.

OCD can't create irritation if you already don't find it irritating

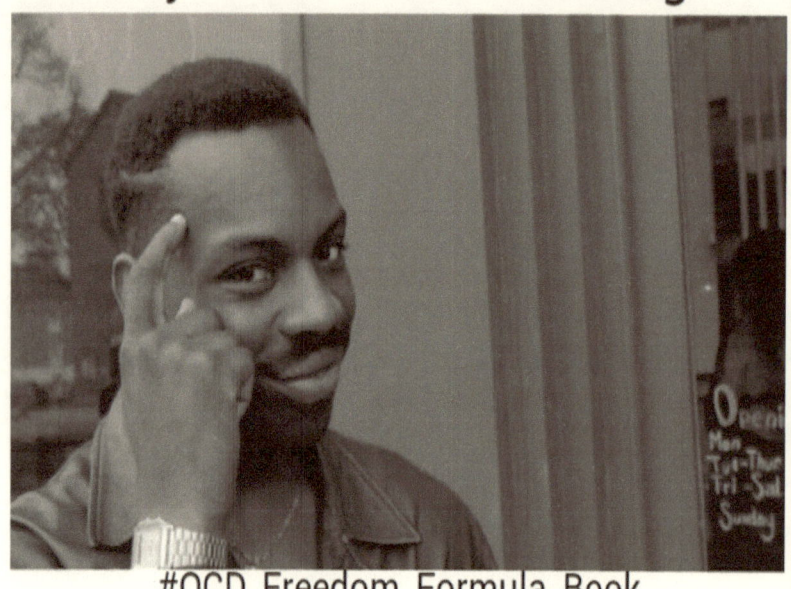

#OCD_Freedom_Formula_Book

APPLICATION OF MECHANISM

UNIT 4

SUMMARIZATION OF THE PROCESS

CHAPTER 21

THE BLUEPRINT

This chapter is presented so you don't get overwhelmed and have a clear direction of what needs to be done.

And yeah I suppose you have finished the previous chapters, if not I request you to do the same otherwise this chapter will be in vain for you.

EACH AND EVERY SECTION OF THE BOOK IS RELATED, LEAVING ANY PART; YOU WILL BE DELAYING YOUR OWN PROCESS OF HEALING.

So, without any further ado let's summarize the process:

1st: First take a leave for a month, where you are free of any external stress.

2nd: Do something fun, something that you enjoy; in that month do something that gives you genuine joy, and makes you forget your worries. Leave all the stressful stuff.

*note: if you can't do the first two part, just see that you minimize your external stress as much as possible, and try to do something that you enjoy even if it's for half an hour.

3rd: Follow the **God Mindset** whenever you have OCD, recite it. With time it will get internalised. This is not something you do for a little while and forget. Though it is mentioned as 3rd for clarity of steps, this is to be done always. This is your main weapon.

4th: Get past your first critical stage. With a fun lifestyle and God mindset in hand, don't do what your OCD wants you to do. Like for example if you have a habit of arranging a shelf, don't do it. And if it's some kind of irritating thought let it come, but you don't think consciously. You accept it, don't resist it. Just take OCD as normal for you now, accept it. Ironically, you actually start to feel better that way.

And yeah on the process of getting past your first critical stage your OCD might go higher, but after a point, it will drop abruptly, if you follow the process dedicatedly. [refer chapter "**Fluctuations and Critical Points**"]

5th: Whenever you hit the normal zone, note down your realization in your journal with the date. You will use this journal as a proof whenever your mind tries to make you believe the bullshit in OCD zone.

6th: You will be fluctuating from normal to OCD to normal zone......but with time when you start hitting more normal zones, you will eventually get healed. So, don't panic from normal zone if you start hitting OCD zone again, accept it even if it comes, and accept the fluctuation. And eventually after some fluctuations you will achieve healed stage. After all it's a part of the process.

So, here you go.

All you need to do now is to follow the process dedicatedly.

CHAPTER 22

FINDING YOUR PASSION

Following I have set up some questions, answering the below questions should help you to realize your passion and dreams and what you actually love doing.

So here goes the questions:

1. **What's that activity, or hobby or time pass that dominates a significant amount of your free time?**

   Explanation:

   Suppose you might think I watch YouTube in my free time. How can YouTube be my passion?

   Don't be like this. Dig deeper, what's in YouTube you often end up searching. Is it about fitness, music or movies or anything else? YouTube is just a medium and the main thing is what you end up searching there most of the time.

   Suppose you always end up listening to music on YouTube, and it takes the maximum amount of your free time. And you might be like how can these be my passion, I cannot sing.

   Maybe true but there are so many things that can be done regarding music: sound engineer, music producer, playing musical instruments, music critic etc....

Or maybe any other hobby or activity like: singing, dancing, sports, reading etc.

World is full of opportunity, you just have to know where to look at.

2. **If you had an unlimited amount of money, what would you do every day?**

3. **What are your super-powers?**

Explanation: When I say super-power what I mean is, what is that thing or unique quality you have that's very special to you a.k.a your natural talent. It's so natural that you don't even realize it. Yeah, sometimes we tend to ignore the natural gifts we have. Because that particular thing is so natural, we don't even pay attention and that quality might be an unconventional one. But quality is quality.

People who are good at speaking, they become a speaker and pursue their passion, or people who are good at math become mathematician e.g.: Albert Einstein was good at math and science and later he became one of the best scientists to take birth on this planet.

You probably got the gist of what I am trying to explain.

4. **What are you interested in?**

Explanation: Interest has a huge contribution in a way that it helps you to build your skill on certain things you are interested at. If you are interested in something it's easy for you to practise that thing for long. You don't get bored easily. Suppose you are interested at playing the guitar, you might not be naturally gifted at guitar skills. But with interest, you practise consistently and you master it anyway.

*the combination of interest and super-power(natural talent) is very lethal. For example, Albert Einstein pursued to become scientist and mathematician at which he had natural talent and also interest at; Lionel Messi became one of the world's best in the field of football which he had interest and also was talented at. Even though the combination of interest and super-power(natural talent) is very lethal but still interest and love for something alone can make you go a long way, Helen Keller can be cited as an example, she was blind-deaf who became a prominent writer in her later years. It's obvious it was not her natural talent but her love and interest in writing took her a long way.

5. **What do you do when you procrastinate? This is important because that particular thing you procrastinate on is probably what you find enjoyable and are attracted to. An author once said : "What you do when you procrastinate is probably what you should be doing all your life."**

6. **If you were guaranteed to succeed at anything but only had one year to live, what would you do?**

Make a list of answers for each question, and the particular thing that comes quite common to most of these questions is probably what you are mostly passionate about.

CHAPTER 23

CORE MINDSETS

Core Mindsets are basically the summarization of all the mindsets mentioned in this book other than the "**GOD Mindset**" and also few extra bonus mindsets.

So, that you don't have to search the whole book for finding your particular favourable and helpful core mindset.

This is the chapter which is the culmination of all those mindsets.

So let's get with it:-

- **"You can only control your mind, by not controlling it"** - more you try to control your mind, more it will fuck you up. If you don't try to control it and let it flow, it will eventually settle. Thus, the secret to controlling your mind is actually not controlling it, ironic right.

- **"Whatever negative is coming to your mind is bullshit, no matter how sensible or rational it seems"**- This holds so true for people who are in OCD. I am very sure sometimes a negative thought comes, and you start believing it. For example, my negative thoughts in OCD were like you will always be miserable, you are hopeless and stuff like that and I actually started believing it. Later, when I was in a healing phase, I realized that it was a bullshit move from my side to believe the negative. It's not 'when people tell you hopeless, or you feel like hopeless' matters, it's only when you start believing yourself as hopeless, you actually start behaving as hopeless. Same for other stuffs. So, never believe any negative thought. If the feeling or the thought coming subconsciously it's okay, don't resist it, accept it, let it come.

Accept it, but don't believe it.

You are in a mental state where comprehending and understanding a situation, a thinking is almost 90% wrong, depending on how serious your OCD is.

The negative self-thought might seem true but it's not. It's just not.

Again *any* negative, by *any* I mean *any any any any any any* single fucking dime of negative is bullshit – thought or feeling whatever no matter how rational and sensible it seems.

- **"Don't try to control or pay attention to the subconscious, just monitor the conscious part and subconscious will automatically change with time."**

- **"OCD feeds on fear, which is irrational. The lesser you fear OCD, the weaker it gets."** – The fact that you fear OCD gives it more power, after coming out of it you will realize it had no power all along. Only the illusion of power. It was only your fear that gave it more power. That's why I say don't fear OCD, make peace with OCD, accept it.

  As you continue with the process laid out in this book, you hit many normal zones; with each hit of normal zone, your fear for OCD will automatically decrease even it is 1%. And as you start to hit more normal zones, your fear will decrease more and you will gradually start to realize the illusion for what it actually is.

- **"Life is an adventure"** – This mindset can be used to cut all the people issue, upset over petty stuff & noises:

  The truth is everything is temporary, as time goes, what people say or think, things happened regarding your relationship everything, everyone will go, everything is so temporary, why are you crying, why are you stressing about it, everything is temporary, why are you stressing about temporary stuff, your girlfriend/boyfriend dumped you. You still have so many years left, it's just a part of a few beginning chapters of your life, there are so many chapters left, so why are you crying over the first few chapters, and even it is from the later chapters, there are still many parts left, story has not ended yet; anything bad happened or that might in your life is temporary, life itself is temporary, take life as an adventure, even bad times are fun and even good times are fun, remain unattached to the things that produce negativity in your life, and stop stressing consciously over things that makes you negative (if it is subconscious, that's okay it will come and go). Life is too short, so follow your dreams, do what you love, go to a party, club, dance, sing and don't give a fuck.

- **"You can be happy, even if you have OCD"** – This is a big myth buster. You can be happy with OCD.

  Yeah, you heard that right.

  OCD makes you think that you can't be happy with it and you believe it, and your believe affects your behaviour and you actually become unhappy.

  An illusion your OCD tries to feed you is that you can't be happy with it; the fact that you think and believe you can't be happy with it, makes it harder for you to be happy.

THUS, THE MORE YOU BELIEVE YOUR HAPPINESS IS INDEPENDENT OF OCD, THE MORE EASIER IT WILL BE FOR YOU TO BE HAPPY.

CHAPTER 24

CONCLUSION

Congratulations, and thank yourself for making a decision to getting access to this book.

As I said like million times till now, follow the process diligently and dedicatedly.

And lemme tell you after overcoming this, when you face with other problems of your life it doesn't even affect you. This is probably the worst thing you have ever faced in your life.

You have all the weapons and the instructions of how to use it.

Happiness is everybody's birthright and you my friend through the process will definitely achieve it.

The program is a result of years spent on my trial and error and research on human mind, me myself going through several medications and therapies namely C.B.T, E.R.P etc.... and research on psychology especially on neuroplasticity, all the knowledge and realizations optimized to get the best results.

The only thing left is patience.

I can show the path, but you yourself have to walk. If you follow the process with mindsets and habits and lifestyle I outlined, you will definitely see improvement.

You have to cast the negative aside that your mind is telling you and once again I say all the negatives are bullshit.

Anything that makes you feel bad no matter how rational it seems is bullshit and false.

Anyways have a happy journey through the entire process, it will be one roller coaster ride, where in the end of the ride you will achieve true happiness and freedom.

LETTER FROM THE AUTHOR:

I gave my everything in this book.

To make it as simple and easy for the readers as possible.

To the point and precise.

I want to make a humble request to you, when you start seeing improvements or if you liked or connected with the book.

Please do leave a review or provide a balanced feedback.

This will make other readers know what the book is about and how helpful the book is.

Your rating and feedback will mean a lot to us.

Thanking you in advance
Steven Paul
OCD Survivor

OCD FREEDOM PROGRAM

First of all.

Let me tell you.

This program is not mandatory nor necessary.

The book itself is more than enough.

But sometimes people want more.

They want the process to be faster and smoother.

If that's you.

Than I would like to invite you to join our "OCD Freedom Program"

If you want to join the program there are 3 pre-requisites :

1. You first need to give atleast 3 months to this book dedicatedly; to understand its concepts and see some improvements as a result. After this only if you feel like joining the program, to fasten the process than you can do so.
2. You have to be dedicated and listen to me carefully, having no ego, because the stuff I will be speaking out on will be really deep.
3. And the third thing.

Well.....let's keep it a secret. Will tell you when you join.

To join send an email at: ocdfreedomprogram@gmail.com

And again I state, as I mentioned before this program is not mandatory nor required, its only a supplement to boost the process.

Anyways wish you a healthy transformation.

And get the life, happiness and freedom you always deserved.

May everyone in this world become OCD-Free one day.

Have Patience.

I know the pain, I have been there.

Follow the process dedicatedly.

And you will see light at the end of the tunnel.

Love you all.

Take Care.

URGENT PLEA!

Thank You For Reading My Book!

I really appreciate all of your feedback, and I love hearing what you have to say.

I need your input to make my future books even better.

Please, leave me a helpful review on Amazon letting me know what you thought of the book.

Thank you so much!
Steven Paul